Winter Glow-Winter-Proof Your Skin in 7 Days

By Dr.joshep

Dedication

To everyone embracing their unique beauty, no matter the season. May your glow radiate always.

1. UNDERSTANDING WINTER SKIN CHALLENGES..... 6

2. THE SCIENCE OF HYDRATION: COMBATTING WINTER DRYNESS 10

3. BUILDING THE ULTIMATE WINTER SKINCARE ROUTINE 15

4. KEY INGREDIENTS FOR RADIANT WINTER SKIN . 21

5. DAY 1 - CLEANSING FOR PROTECTION AND BALANCE 26

6. DAY 2 - HYDRATING AND REPLENISHING YOUR SKIN 32

7. DAY 3 - NOURISHING YOUR SKIN FOR BARRIER REPAIR 38

8. DAY 4 - GENTLE EXFOLIATION FOR A RADIANT WINTER GLOW 44

9. DAY 5 - TARGETED TREATMENTS FOR WINTER SKIN CONCERNS 50

10. DAY 6 - CREATING A PROTECTIVE BARRIER FOR WINTER SKIN 56

11. DAY 7 - SUSTAINING YOUR WINTER GLOW 62

12. THE ROLE OF NUTRITION IN SKIN HEALTH 68

13. OVERCOMING COMMON WINTER SKIN ISSUES. 75

14. DIY SKINCARE – AFFORDABLE REMEDIES FOR WINTER 83

15. **MAINTAINING YOUR GLOW BEYOND THE 7-DAY CHALLENGE** 90

Introduction:

Winter brings a serene beauty with its frosty mornings and snow-clad landscapes, but it also ushers in challenges for your skin. Cold winds, low humidity, and indoor heating strip moisture from your skin, leaving it dry, dull, and prone to irritation. The fight against winter skin woes can feel endless, but achieving a luminous, healthy complexion during this season is entirely possible.

"Winter Glow - Winter-Proof Your Skin in 7 Days" is your ultimate guide to unlocking radiant skin, no matter how harsh the season gets. Designed for simplicity and effectiveness, this book provides a 7-day skincare regimen that will transform your skin's texture, hydration, and overall appearance. With practical advice, expert insights, and actionable steps, this guide caters to individuals across all skin types and lifestyles.

Within these pages, you'll uncover:

- The science behind winter skin and why hydration is the cornerstone of any winter skincare regimen.
- A breakdown of essential ingredients to protect, repair, and nourish your skin.
- Daily routines designed to address key skin needs while fitting seamlessly into your schedule.

- Bonus tips on nutrition and lifestyle to enhance your results from the inside out.

Each chapter not only educates but also empowers you to take charge of your skin health. Whether you're battling stubborn dry patches, looking to maintain your summer glow, or simply seeking to understand your skin better, this book is your roadmap to success.

So, get ready to wrap your skin in care and achieve that enviable winter glow. Let's embark on this journey together and prove that winter can be a season for radiant beauty.

***

Understanding Winter Skin Challenges

Winter is a season of contrasts—pristine white landscapes, festive celebrations, and cozy firesides. Yet, beneath this charm lies a hidden adversary for your skin. The colder months test your skin's resilience, and understanding the challenges is the first step toward achieving a radiant winter glow.

The Effects of Winter on Skin

As temperatures drop, so does the humidity in the air. The cold winds and dry indoor heating systems contribute to a significant loss of moisture from the skin. This phenomenon, known as transepidermal water loss (TEWL), weakens the skin's barrier function, leading to dryness, sensitivity, and irritation. The result? Dull, flaky skin that feels tight and uncomfortable.

Common Winter Skin Issues

1. **Dryness and Dehydration**
   The lack of moisture in the air depletes your skin's natural hydration levels, leaving it parched and vulnerable.
2. **Flakiness and Rough Texture**
   Dead skin cells accumulate more during winter, leading to a rough, uneven texture.
3. **Redness and Irritation**
   Sensitive skin becomes more reactive in winter, with redness and irritation becoming frequent companions.

4. **Cracked Lips and Hands**
   Exposed areas like lips and hands are particularly prone to cracking and chapping, often requiring extra care.

Why Winter Skin Needs Special Attention

The skin's lipid barrier acts as its protective shield. In winter, this barrier is compromised by environmental stressors, making it essential to replenish and reinforce its defenses. Without proper care, the skin can become inflamed, exacerbating conditions such as eczema, rosacea, and psoriasis.

The Role of Lifestyle in Winter Skin Health

Beyond environmental factors, our lifestyle choices often intensify winter skin challenges. Long, hot showers might feel soothing but strip the skin of its natural oils. Wearing heavy, non-breathable fabrics can cause friction and irritation, and skipping sunscreen due to fewer sunny days can expose the skin to harmful UV rays.

Key Myths About Winter Skin

1. **Myth:** "My skin doesn't need sunscreen in winter."
   Fact: UV rays can penetrate clouds and reflect off snow, making sunscreen a year-round necessity.
2. **Myth:** "Oily skin doesn't dry out in winter."
   Fact: Even oily skin can become

dehydrated, requiring hydration without overloading on heavy creams.

3. **Myth:** "Drinking water alone can keep my skin hydrated."
Fact: While hydration from within is vital, external care like moisturizing and using occlusive products is equally important.

Preparing Your Skin for Winter

Before diving into the 7-day skincare challenge, it's crucial to set the foundation:

- **Switch to Gentle Cleansers:** Replace harsh foaming cleansers with creamy or hydrating options.
- **Introduce Humidifiers:** Combat indoor dryness by keeping the air around you hydrated.
- **Layer Skincare Products:** Learn the art of layering—from serums to moisturizers—to lock in hydration effectively.
- **Prioritize Lip and Hand Care:** Stock up on nourishing balms and hand creams to shield these areas from the elements.

The Mindset Shift

Winter skincare is not just about addressing problems—it's about embracing the opportunity to pamper and protect your skin. By understanding the challenges and preparing strategically, you'll create a solid foundation for glowing skin all season long.

In the next chapter, we'll explore the science of hydration and how you can harness it to combat winter dryness effectively. Get ready to delve deeper into the journey of achieving your winter glow!

***

The Science of Hydration: Combatting Winter Dryness

Hydration is the cornerstone of healthy, glowing skin, especially during the winter months. While it might seem as simple as applying a moisturizer, effective hydration requires an understanding of how the skin works, the role of water, and the tools needed to maintain moisture balance.

The Skin's Hydration Mechanism

The skin consists of three primary layers:

1. **Epidermis (Outer Layer):** This layer contains the stratum corneum, which acts as a protective barrier and is responsible for retaining water.
2. **Dermis (Middle Layer):** This layer houses collagen, elastin, and hyaluronic acid, which help maintain skin's plumpness and elasticity.
3. **Subcutaneous Layer (Deepest Layer):** Primarily made of fat, this layer provides insulation and energy storage.

In winter, the epidermis suffers the most due to environmental conditions. The stratum corneum loses moisture faster, and without intervention, it can lead to dehydration and a compromised barrier.

Water Content in the Skin

Healthy skin is about 64% water. When hydration levels drop, the skin becomes less effective at defending itself against external irritants. Maintaining this water balance is critical for keeping your skin supple and resilient.

Factors That Cause Winter Dryness

1. **Low Humidity:** Cold air holds less moisture, which leads to increased water loss from the skin.
2. **Indoor Heating:** Central heating systems further deplete moisture levels in the air, creating a drying environment.
3. **Harsh Cleansers:** Using products that strip the skin's natural oils can exacerbate dehydration.
4. **Hot Showers and Baths:** Prolonged exposure to hot water may feel comforting but disrupts the skin's lipid barrier.

Key Ingredients for Hydration

To combat winter dryness, it's essential to incorporate hydrating ingredients into your skincare routine. Let's explore the most effective options:

1. **Hyaluronic Acid (HA):**
   - A powerful humectant that attracts water to the skin, HA can hold up to 1,000 times its weight in water.

- o Best applied on damp skin to maximize its hydrating effects.

2. **Glycerin:**
   - o A common yet effective humectant that draws moisture from the air and locks it into the skin.
   - o Works well in combination with other hydrating ingredients.

3. **Ceramides:**
   - o Lipid molecules that help restore the skin's barrier, preventing water loss.
   - o Particularly useful for sensitive or eczema-prone skin.

4. **Squalane:**
   - o Mimics the skin's natural oils, providing lightweight hydration and reinforcing the lipid barrier.

5. **Occlusives:**
   - o Ingredients like petrolatum, shea butter, and beeswax form a protective layer to seal in moisture.
   - o Best used as a final step in your routine, especially at night.

Building a Hydration-Focused Routine

Achieving optimal hydration requires a consistent routine tailored to winter's demands.

1. **Morning Routine:**
   - o **Cleanser:** Use a gentle, hydrating cleanser to remove impurities without stripping natural oils.
   - o **Toner or Mist:** Apply a hydrating toner or mist to prep the skin.

- o **Serum:** Opt for a hyaluronic acid or glycerin-based serum for a hydration boost.
  - o **Moisturizer:** Seal in hydration with a ceramide-rich moisturizer.
  - o **Sunscreen:** Never skip sunscreen, even on cloudy days.

2. **Evening Routine:**
   - o **Double Cleansing:** If wearing makeup, start with an oil-based cleanser, followed by a gentle hydrating cleanser.
   - o **Exfoliation (2-3 times a week):** Use a mild chemical exfoliant to remove dead skin cells and improve absorption.
   - o **Hydrating Serum:** Reapply your serum to replenish moisture overnight.
   - o **Night Cream:** Choose a heavier occlusive cream or sleeping mask to lock in hydration.

Lifestyle Tips for Hydration

1. **Drink Water Regularly:** While external hydration is vital, internal hydration is equally important. Aim for at least 2 liters daily.
2. **Use a Humidifier:** Adding moisture to indoor air can significantly reduce dryness.
3. **Avoid Overheating Indoors:** Keep your thermostat at a moderate level to prevent excessive moisture loss.
4. **Wear Protective Clothing:** Scarves, gloves, and hats can shield your skin from harsh winds.

Signs of Properly Hydrated Skin

When your skin is well-hydrated, it appears plump, smooth, and radiant. Fine lines caused by dehydration diminish, and the skin feels comfortable and balanced rather than tight or flaky.

Hydration is not just a seasonal requirement but a year-round commitment. However, winter demands extra vigilance to counteract the drying effects of the environment. With the right products, routine, and lifestyle adjustments, your skin can thrive even in the harshest conditions.

In the next chapter, we'll focus on creating a winter skincare routine tailored to your needs, ensuring every step contributes to your journey toward the perfect winter glow.

***

Building the Ultimate Winter Skincare Routine

A skincare routine is not just a daily habit—it's an investment in the health and appearance of your skin. During winter, the stakes are higher as cold weather, harsh winds, and indoor heating work together to strip your skin of moisture and vitality. This chapter will guide you through crafting a winter skincare routine that addresses these challenges head-on.

Understanding the Importance of Routine

Skincare is most effective when it follows a consistent structure. Each step in your routine serves a purpose, from cleansing to treating and protecting your skin. A winter skincare routine should prioritize hydration, protection, and repair to combat the season's unique stressors.

Step-by-Step Guide to Your Winter Skincare Routine

Morning Routine: Prepping Your Skin for the Day

1. **Gentle Cleansing**
   - **Why It Matters:** Overnight, your skin accumulates sweat, oils, and environmental pollutants. A gentle cleanse prepares your skin for the day without disrupting its moisture barrier.
   - **Best Products:** Cream or gel-based cleansers that are free of sulfates.
2. **Hydrating Toner or Essence**
   - **Why It Matters:** Toners help balance the skin's pH while providing an additional layer of hydration.
   - **Best Ingredients:** Aloe vera, glycerin, or panthenol for a soothing effect.
3. **Hydrating Serum**
   - **Why It Matters:** Serums are concentrated treatments that penetrate deeper into the skin. A hydrating serum ensures moisture reaches the dermis.
   - **Best Ingredients:** Hyaluronic acid, niacinamide, and vitamin B5.
4. **Moisturizer**
   - **Why It Matters:** A good moisturizer locks in the hydration from your serum and forms a protective barrier.
   - **Best Products:** Ceramide-rich creams or those with natural oils like jojoba or squalane.

5. **Sunscreen**
   - o **Why It Matters:** UV rays can penetrate clouds and reflect off snow, causing skin damage even in winter.
   - o **Best Products:** Broad-spectrum SPF 30 or higher, ideally with added antioxidants.

Evening Routine: Repair and Replenish

1. **Double Cleansing**
   - o **Why It Matters:** Removes makeup, sunscreen, and impurities from the day while ensuring your skin is clean without being stripped of its natural oils.
   - o **How to Do It:** Start with an oil-based cleanser to break down makeup and follow with a gentle hydrating cleanser.
2. **Exfoliation (2-3 Times Per Week)**
   - o **Why It Matters:** Exfoliation removes dead skin cells, improves product absorption, and prevents flaky skin.
   - o **Best Options:** Gentle chemical exfoliants like lactic acid or mandelic acid, which are less likely to irritate winter skin.
3. **Treatment Serums**
   - o **Why It Matters:** Target specific skin concerns like hyperpigmentation, fine lines, or dehydration.
   - o **Best Ingredients:** Retinol for repair, peptides for skin renewal, or

hydrating serums for added moisture.

4. **Night Cream or Sleeping Mask**
   - **Why It Matters:** Nighttime is when your skin repairs itself. A richer cream or mask can provide deeper hydration and nourishment.
   - **Best Products:** Formulas with shea butter, ceramides, or hyaluronic acid.
5. **Lip Balm and Hand Cream**
   - **Why It Matters:** These exposed areas need extra care to prevent chapping and cracking.

Weekly Add-Ons to Boost Results

1. **Face Masks (Once or Twice a Week)**
   - **Hydrating Masks:** Packed with ingredients like aloe vera or hyaluronic acid for intense hydration.
   - **Nourishing Masks:** Include oils or ceramides to repair the skin barrier.
2. **Eye Cream or Mask**
   - Focus on reducing puffiness, dark circles, and dryness around the eyes.

Customizing Your Routine by Skin Type

1. **Dry Skin**
   - Focus on rich, occlusive moisturizers and limit exfoliation to once a week.
   - Incorporate face oils like rosehip or argan oil for added nourishment.
2. **Oily or Combination Skin**
   - Use lightweight, non-comedogenic moisturizers and hydrating serums.
   - Avoid overly rich creams that may clog pores.
3. **Sensitive Skin**
   - Opt for fragrance-free products and patch test new items.
   - Use calming ingredients like chamomile, centella asiatica, or colloidal oatmeal.

Protecting Your Skin Beyond Products

1. **Layer Your Clothing:** Wear breathable fabrics and use scarves to shield your face from windburn.
2. **Manage Indoor Heating:** Keep your thermostat moderate and use a humidifier to maintain indoor moisture.
3. **Stay Hydrated:** Drink plenty of water and include hydrating foods like cucumber, oranges, and watermelon in your diet.

A well-structured winter skincare routine doesn't just protect your skin—it enhances its resilience, ensuring you glow throughout the season. In the next chapter, we'll explore the key ingredients that make a real difference in winter skincare, helping you make informed choices tailored to your needs.

***

Key Ingredients for Radiant Winter Skin

Winter skincare hinges on the quality of the ingredients you incorporate into your routine. The right ingredients can hydrate, protect, and repair your skin, giving it the resilience to combat the harshness of the season. This chapter dives into the essential components of effective winter skincare, their benefits, and how to choose products that work best for you.

The Three Pillars of Winter Skincare Ingredients

1. **Humectants**
   - **Function:** Attract moisture from the environment or deeper layers of the skin to the surface, keeping your skin hydrated.
   - **Key Ingredients:** Hyaluronic acid, glycerin, aloe vera, panthenol.
2. **Emollients**
   - **Function:** Fill in the gaps between skin cells, smoothing and softening rough patches.
   - **Key Ingredients:** Squalane, fatty acids, shea butter, jojoba oil, ceramides.
3. **Occlusives**
   - **Function:** Create a protective barrier on the skin to lock in moisture and prevent water loss.
   - **Key Ingredients:** Petrolatum, beeswax, lanolin, cocoa butter.

Top Ingredients to Look for in Winter Skincare

1. **Hyaluronic Acid (HA)**
   - **Why It's Essential:** Known for its unparalleled ability to retain water, HA deeply hydrates and plumps the skin.
   - **How to Use:** Apply on damp skin and follow with a moisturizer to lock in the hydration.
2. **Ceramides**
   - **Why It's Essential:** These lipids restore the skin's barrier function, reducing dryness and sensitivity.
   - **Best For:** All skin types, especially dry or sensitive skin.
3. **Squalane**
   - **Why It's Essential:** A lightweight oil that mimics the skin's natural sebum, squalane provides moisture without feeling greasy.
   - **Best For:** Oily or combination skin prone to dehydration.
4. **Glycerin**
   - **Why It's Essential:** A versatile humectant, glycerin draws moisture to the skin and improves hydration at the surface level.
   - **How to Use:** Commonly found in cleansers, serums, and moisturizers.
5. **Shea Butter**
   - **Why It's Essential:** Rich in fatty acids and vitamins, shea butter nourishes and protects the skin from harsh elements.
   - **Best For:** Dry and flaky skin.
6. **Niacinamide (Vitamin B3)**

- o **Why It's Essential:** This multi-tasking ingredient improves hydration, reduces redness, and strengthens the skin's barrier.
- o **Best For:** All skin types, especially those with redness or irritation.

7. **Aloe Vera**
- o **Why It's Essential:** A natural humectant with soothing properties, aloe vera calms irritated or inflamed skin while hydrating.
- o **Best For:** Sensitive or irritated skin.

8. **Vitamin E**
- o **Why It's Essential:** A powerful antioxidant that helps neutralize free radicals and supports skin repair.
- o **Best For:** Use in combination with other antioxidants like Vitamin C for added benefits.

9. **Lactic Acid**
- o **Why It's Essential:** A gentle exfoliant that removes dead skin cells while retaining moisture.
- o **Best For:** Those dealing with dull, flaky winter skin.

10. **Petrolatum**
- o **Why It's Essential:** A heavy-duty occlusive that locks in moisture and heals dry, cracked skin.
- o **Best For:** Targeted areas like hands, elbows, and heels.

How to Identify Quality Products

1. **Check the Ingredient Order:** Ingredients are listed by concentration. Ensure key ingredients like hyaluronic acid or ceramides are listed near the top.
2. **Look for Fragrance-Free Options:** Fragrance can irritate sensitive skin, especially in winter.
3. **Avoid Harsh Alcohols:** Ingredients like denatured alcohol can dry out the skin; opt for fatty alcohols like cetyl alcohol instead.
4. **Patch Test New Products:** Always test new products on a small area to prevent potential reactions.

Layering Ingredients for Maximum Benefits

The effectiveness of your winter skincare routine depends on the order in which products are applied. Follow this layering strategy:

1. Start with lighter, water-based products like toners and serums.
2. Follow with heavier, oil-based moisturizers and occlusives.
3. Always finish with sunscreen during the day to protect from UV rays.

DIY Skincare Using Winter-Friendly Ingredients

1. **Hydrating Face Mask:**
   - **Ingredients:** 2 tbsp aloe vera gel, 1 tsp honey, a few drops of rosehip oil.
   - **How to Use:** Mix and apply to the face. Leave on for 15 minutes, then rinse with lukewarm water.
2. **Lip Balm:**
   - **Ingredients:** 1 tbsp shea butter, 1 tsp beeswax, 1 tsp coconut oil.
   - **How to Use:** Melt the ingredients together, pour into a container, and let cool.
3. **Hand Cream:**
   - **Ingredients:** 2 tbsp cocoa butter, 1 tbsp olive oil, 1 tsp glycerin.
   - **How to Use:** Blend and store in a small jar for daily use.

Conclusion

The right ingredients are the backbone of any effective winter skincare routine. By understanding their functions and selecting products tailored to your needs, you can build a regimen that keeps your skin hydrated, healthy, and glowing. In the next chapter, we'll dive into the first day of the 7-day winter-proof skincare challenge, starting with the art of cleansing for protection.

***

Day 1 - Cleansing for Protection and Balance

The foundation of any skincare routine lies in cleansing. It's the first step that sets the tone for how well your skin absorbs and benefits from the products that follow. During winter, cleansing takes on an added dimension—not only must it remove impurities, but it must also protect and preserve the skin's natural moisture barrier.

Why Cleansing Is Crucial in Winter

Cleansing removes dirt, oil, sweat, and pollutants that accumulate on your skin throughout the day or night. However, winter's dry air and harsh conditions can make the skin more vulnerable to stripping and irritation, especially when using the wrong cleansers.

A winter-appropriate cleanser should:

1. Remove impurities without over-drying the skin.
2. Support hydration by retaining the skin's natural oils.
3. Be gentle enough to avoid disrupting the protective barrier.

Choosing the Right Cleanser for Winter

Types of Cleansers to Consider

1. **Cream Cleansers**
   - **Description:** Rich and moisturizing, cream cleansers are ideal for dry and sensitive skin.
   - **Best For:** Dry, mature, or sensitive skin types.
   - **Key Ingredients:** Ceramides, glycerin, and shea butter.
2. **Gel Cleansers**
   - **Description:** Lightweight and refreshing, gel cleansers are effective at removing impurities without leaving a heavy residue.
   - **Best For:** Oily or combination skin.
   - **Key Ingredients:** Aloe vera, chamomile, or cucumber extract.
3. **Oil Cleansers**
   - **Description:** Excellent for breaking down makeup and sunscreen, oil cleansers also provide nourishment during the cleansing process.
   - **Best For:** All skin types, especially dry or sensitive skin.
   - **Key Ingredients:** Jojoba oil, argan oil, or sunflower seed oil.
4. **Micellar Water**
   - **Description:** A no-rinse option that uses micelles to lift away dirt and oil while being gentle on the skin.
   - **Best For:** Quick cleansing or sensitive skin.

o **Key Ingredients:** Glycerin and soothing botanical extracts.

What to Avoid

- **Harsh Sulfates:** Ingredients like sodium lauryl sulfate can strip your skin of essential oils.
- **Alcohol-Based Products:** These can exacerbate dryness and irritation.
- **Fragrance and Dyes:** Opt for fragrance-free formulations to reduce the risk of sensitivity.

Cleansing Routine for Morning and Night

Morning Routine: Preparing Your Skin for the Day

1. **Start with Lukewarm Water**
   o Avoid hot water as it can strip the skin of its natural oils.
2. **Use a Gentle Cleanser**
   o Apply a small amount of your winter-friendly cleanser to damp skin. Massage in circular motions to remove sweat and sebum.
3. **Rinse Thoroughly**
   o Ensure all product is removed to avoid residue that can clog pores or irritate the skin.
4. **Pat Dry with a Soft Towel**

- o Avoid rubbing the skin to prevent micro-tears or irritation.

Night Routine: Reset and Repair

1. **Double Cleansing**
   - o Begin with an oil-based cleanser to remove makeup and sunscreen. Follow with a gentle cleanser to ensure all impurities are lifted.
2. **Focus on Problem Areas**
   - o Pay extra attention to areas prone to dryness or congestion, such as around the nose and chin.
3. **Follow Immediately with Hydration**
   - o Apply a hydrating toner or serum while the skin is still damp to lock in moisture.

Tips for Enhancing Your Cleansing Routine

1. **Use a Cleansing Brush or Cloth**
   - o These tools can help exfoliate gently, improving circulation and product absorption.
   - o Avoid overusing them, as excessive exfoliation can damage the barrier.
2. **Incorporate a Weekly Steam Session**
   - o Fill a bowl with hot water, add a few drops of essential oils like lavender or eucalyptus, and steam your face for 5-10 minutes. This opens pores and enhances the efficacy of your cleanser.

3. **Don't Skip Cleansing Even on No-Makeup Days**
   o Dirt, sweat, and environmental pollutants still accumulate and need to be removed daily.

DIY Cleansing Recipes for Winter

1. **Honey and Milk Cleanser**
   o **Ingredients:** 1 tbsp raw honey, 2 tbsp milk.
   o **How to Use:** Mix and massage onto your skin. Rinse with lukewarm water. This cleanser soothes and hydrates.
2. **Oatmeal Cleanser**
   o **Ingredients:** 1 tbsp ground oats, 1 tsp almond oil, water.
   o **How to Use:** Create a paste and gently scrub onto damp skin. This acts as a cleanser and exfoliant.

Signs of Effective Cleansing

- Your skin feels clean but not tight or dry.
- No residue or makeup remains on the skin.
- Your skin appears refreshed and ready for the next step in your routine.

Conclusion

Day 1 of your winter-proof skincare journey is about mastering the art of cleansing. With the right products, techniques, and consistency, this foundational step will prepare your skin to absorb the benefits of hydration and nourishment in the days ahead.

In the next chapter, we'll focus on Day 2 of the 7-day plan—hydrating and replenishing your skin to maintain its glow through the season.

***

Day 2 - Hydrating and Replenishing Your Skin

Hydration is the cornerstone of healthy, glowing skin, especially during winter. While cleansing ensures your skin is free from impurities, hydration replenishes the moisture lost to cold winds, dry air, and indoor heating. This chapter explores how to restore and maintain optimal hydration levels, ensuring your skin remains supple and resilient throughout the season.

Why Hydration Matters in Winter

The skin's outermost layer, the stratum corneum, serves as a barrier to retain moisture and protect against environmental aggressors. In winter, this barrier is compromised, leading to transepidermal water loss (TEWL). Hydrating and replenishing the skin restores this barrier, preventing dryness, flaking, and irritation.

Hydration Essentials for All Skin Types

1. **Humectants: Attracting Water**
   - **How They Work:** Humectants draw moisture to the skin, either from the environment or deeper layers.

- o **Key Ingredients:** Hyaluronic acid, glycerin, aloe vera, urea.
2. **Emollients: Smoothing and Softening**
   - o **How They Work:** Emollients fill in gaps between skin cells, making the skin smoother and softer.
   - o **Key Ingredients:** Squalane, fatty acids, shea butter, ceramides.
3. **Occlusives: Sealing in Moisture**
   - o **How They Work:** Occlusives form a barrier on the skin, preventing moisture from escaping.
   - o **Key Ingredients:** Petrolatum, beeswax, lanolin, cocoa butter.

Steps for Deep Hydration

Morning Hydration Routine

1. **Hydrating Toner or Essence**
   - o **Why It's Important:** Prepares the skin for better absorption of subsequent products.
   - o **How to Use:** Apply with hands or a cotton pad, pressing gently into the skin.
2. **Hydrating Serum**
   - o **Focus Ingredients:** Hyaluronic acid for moisture retention and niacinamide for barrier strengthening.
   - o **How to Use:** Use 2-3 drops and press into damp skin for maximum absorption.

o
3. **Moisturizer**
    - o **What to Look For:** A lightweight but nourishing formula that doesn't feel heavy.
    - o **Key Ingredients:** Ceramides and natural oils.
4. **Sunscreen**
    - o **Why It's Necessary:** Even in winter, UV rays can dehydrate and damage your skin.

Evening Hydration Routine

1. **Layer Your Serums**
    - o Use multiple serums if necessary: start with the lightest, water-based formulas.
2. **Use a Night Cream or Sleeping Mask**
    - o Opt for products enriched with occlusives like shea butter to lock in hydration overnight.
3. **Don't Forget Targeted Areas**
    - o Use lip balms with beeswax or petroleum jelly and hand creams with glycerin.

The Role of Diet in Skin Hydration

Hydrating your skin isn't just about topical products—it also involves internal hydration through your diet and water intake.

1. **Hydration from Within**
   - Drink at least 2 liters of water daily to keep skin cells hydrated.
   - Include herbal teas like chamomile or green tea for antioxidants and hydration.
2. **Skin-Boosting Foods**
   - **High-Water Content Foods:** Watermelon, cucumber, oranges.
   - **Omega-3 Rich Foods:** Salmon, flaxseeds, walnuts for skin barrier repair.
   - **Antioxidant-Rich Foods:** Berries, spinach, and sweet potatoes for combating oxidative stress.

DIY Hydrating Treatments for Winter

1. **Hyaluronic Acid Mist**
   - **Ingredients:** 1 tsp hyaluronic acid powder, 1 cup distilled water.
   - **How to Use:** Store in a spray bottle and mist throughout the day for instant hydration.
2. **Honey and Yogurt Mask**
   - **Ingredients:** 1 tbsp honey, 2 tbsp plain yogurt.
   - **How to Use:** Mix, apply to your face, and leave for 15 minutes before rinsing.
3. **Cucumber and Aloe Vera Gel Pack**
   - **Ingredients:** 2 tbsp aloe vera gel, 1 tbsp cucumber juice.
   - **How to Use:** Mix and apply as a hydrating pack for 20 minutes.

How to Tell if Your Skin is Properly Hydrated

1. **Plumpness and Elasticity:** Hydrated skin appears bouncy and firm to the touch.
2. **Smooth Texture:** A lack of rough patches or flakiness indicates adequate hydration.
3. **Radiance:** Properly hydrated skin glows naturally, even without makeup.
4. **Comfort:** No tightness or irritation, even in dry indoor conditions.

Avoiding Hydration Mistakes

1. **Skipping Moisturizer:** Hydration serums need to be sealed in with a moisturizer to prevent evaporation.
2. **Using Hot Water:** Hot showers can strip your skin of its natural oils, leading to dehydration.
3. **Neglecting Sunscreen:** UV rays deplete skin hydration, making sunscreen a non-negotiable.

Conclusion

Day 2 of your winter skincare challenge is all about infusing your skin with moisture and replenishing its hydration levels. By choosing the right ingredients, following a thoughtful routine, and maintaining healthy habits, you can counteract the drying effects of winter.

In the next chapter, we'll explore Day 3— nourishing your skin with the right nutrients to repair and strengthen your barrier.

***

Day 3 - Nourishing Your Skin for Barrier Repair

Nourishing your skin is a critical step in any skincare regimen, particularly during winter. While hydration replenishes moisture, nourishment provides the essential nutrients your skin needs to repair, regenerate, and strengthen its natural barrier. In this chapter, we focus on the importance of skin nourishment, the best ingredients to use, and techniques to ensure your skin remains healthy and resilient.

The Role of Skin Nourishment

The skin barrier, primarily composed of lipids, serves as the first line of defense against environmental stressors and water loss. When this barrier is compromised, the skin becomes prone to dryness, irritation, and sensitivity. Proper nourishment rebuilds this barrier, ensuring it can:

1. Retain moisture effectively.
2. Protect against pollutants and allergens.
3. Support natural healing processes.

Key Nutrients for Skin Nourishment

1. **Fatty Acids**
   - **Role:** Strengthen the lipid layer of the skin barrier.

- o **Sources:** Omega-3 and omega-6 fatty acids, found in products with rosehip oil, sunflower oil, and shea butter.

2. **Vitamins**
   - o **Vitamin E:** Protects against free radicals and strengthens the skin barrier.
   - o **Vitamin C:** Boosts collagen production and brightens the skin.
   - o **Vitamin A (Retinoids):** Promotes cell turnover and repair.

3. **Antioxidants**
   - o **Role:** Neutralize free radicals caused by environmental aggressors.
   - o **Sources:** Green tea extract, resveratrol, niacinamide.

4. **Amino Acids**
   - o **Role:** Support the production of proteins like collagen and elastin for firm, healthy skin.
   - o **Sources:** Silk proteins, peptides, and natural amino acids in skincare.

5. **Hydrating Oils**
   - o **Role:** Provide deep nourishment while sealing in moisture.
   - o **Sources:** Argan oil, jojoba oil, and avocado oil.

How to Incorporate Nourishment into Your Routine

Morning Routine

1. **Nourishing Serum:**
   - Choose a serum with niacinamide or Vitamin C for antioxidant protection.
2. **Moisturizer with Lipid-Rich Ingredients:**
   - Opt for creams containing ceramides or fatty acids to rebuild the barrier.
3. **Sunscreen:**
   - Use a broad-spectrum sunscreen enriched with antioxidants to nourish and protect.

Evening Routine

1. **Nourishing Oil:**
   - After applying your serum, layer a facial oil like rosehip or argan oil to lock in nutrients.
2. **Overnight Repair Cream:**
   - Use a thick, occlusive cream that contains ingredients like Vitamin E or peptides.
3. **Targeted Treatments:**
   - Apply retinoids or night serums with active ingredients to promote cell repair while you sleep.

DIY Recipes for Skin Nourishment

1. **Barrier Repair Mask**
   - **Ingredients:** 1 tbsp avocado, 1 tsp honey, a few drops of olive oil.
   - **How to Use:** Mix into a paste and apply to clean skin. Leave for 15 minutes before rinsing.
2. **Vitamin E Oil Blend**
   - **Ingredients:** 2 capsules of Vitamin E, 1 tbsp jojoba oil, 1 tsp almond oil.
   - **How to Use:** Massage into the skin as the last step of your evening routine.
3. **Collagen-Boosting Serum**
   - **Ingredients:** 1 tsp aloe vera gel, 1 tsp rosehip oil, 2 drops of frankincense essential oil.
   - **How to Use:** Apply to damp skin before moisturizer.

Foods for Skin Nourishment

1. **Healthy Fats:**
   - Include foods like salmon, avocados, and nuts to provide essential fatty acids.
2. **Vitamin-Rich Produce:**
   - Bright-colored vegetables like carrots and bell peppers are rich in Vitamins A and C.
3. **Hydrating Options:**
   - Water-rich foods like cucumbers, tomatoes, and leafy greens help maintain moisture levels.
4. **Antioxidant Powerhouses:**

- o Blueberries, green tea, and dark chocolate protect against oxidative stress.

Tips for Maximizing Skin Nourishment

1. **Don't Skip Moisturizer After Cleansing:**
   - o Apply products immediately after cleansing to trap hydration and deliver nutrients effectively.
2. **Layer Products Correctly:**
   - o Start with lighter, water-based serums and layer richer oils or creams on top.
3. **Use Products Consistently:**
   - o Barrier repair takes time. Stick to your routine for visible results.
4. **Avoid Over-Exfoliating:**
   - o Too much exfoliation can strip the skin of essential lipids, negating nourishment efforts.

Signs Your Skin Is Properly Nourished

1. **Smooth Texture:** No rough patches or flaking.
2. **Improved Resilience:** Less sensitivity to cold and environmental stressors.
3. **Healthy Glow:** A radiant, plump appearance.
4. **Even Tone:** Fewer signs of redness or irritation.

Conclusion

Day 3 of your winter-proof skincare challenge focuses on providing your skin with the nourishment it needs to heal and thrive. By using nutrient-rich ingredients, both topically and through your diet, you can repair your skin barrier and prepare it for the harsher conditions ahead.

In the next chapter, we'll tackle Day 4, where we explore exfoliation and how to do it gently to maintain your winter glow.

***

Day 4 - Gentle Exfoliation for a Radiant Winter Glow

Exfoliation is essential for healthy skin, removing dead skin cells to reveal the fresh, radiant layer underneath. However, winter calls for a gentler approach to avoid over-stripping and damaging your skin's delicate barrier. In this chapter, we'll dive into why exfoliation is crucial, how to do it safely during colder months, and the best methods to achieve a luminous winter glow.

Why Exfoliation Matters

Dead skin cells accumulate over time, creating a dull complexion and hindering the absorption of skincare products. Gentle exfoliation:

1. Improves texture by removing flaky patches.
2. Enhances product penetration for better results.
3. Encourages cell turnover, which slows down during winter.

Types of Exfoliation

1. **Physical Exfoliation**
   - o **How It Works:** Uses scrubs or brushes to manually remove dead skin cells.
   - o **Best For:** Normal to oily skin types.
   - o **Caution:** Avoid harsh scrubs with large, jagged particles like apricot pits, which can cause microtears.
2. **Chemical Exfoliation**
   - o **How It Works:** Uses acids or enzymes to dissolve dead skin cells.
   - o **Best For:** Dry, sensitive, or combination skin types.
   - o **Common Ingredients:**
     - **AHAs (Alpha Hydroxy Acids):** Glycolic acid, lactic acid—ideal for dry skin.
     - **BHAs (Beta Hydroxy Acids):** Salicylic acid—perfect for oily or acne-prone skin.
     - **Enzymes:** Derived from fruits like papaya or pineapple for the gentlest exfoliation.
3. **Exfoliating Tools**
   - o **Examples:** Soft-bristle brushes, konjac sponges, or silicone cleansing devices.
   - o **Caution:** Use sparingly to avoid irritation.

How to Exfoliate Safely in Winter

1. **Start Slow**
   - Limit exfoliation to 1-2 times per week, especially if you have sensitive skin.
2. **Choose the Right Product**
   - Opt for gentler formulas with soothing ingredients like aloe vera or chamomile.
3. **Time It Right**
   - Exfoliate at night to avoid immediate sun exposure, which can increase sensitivity.
4. **Follow Up with Hydration**
   - Always moisturize after exfoliating to replenish the skin barrier.
5. **Patch Test**
   - Test new exfoliants on a small area before full application to ensure compatibility.

Exfoliation Routine for Different Skin Types

Dry Skin

- **Product:** Lactic acid-based exfoliants or enzyme masks.
- **Frequency:** Once a week.
- **Tips:** Follow with a thick moisturizer containing ceramides.

Oily or Acne-Prone Skin

- **Product:** Salicylic acid or gentle scrubs with fine particles.
- **Frequency:** 2-3 times a week.
- **Tips:** Focus on areas prone to congestion, such as the T-zone.

Sensitive Skin

- **Product:** Enzyme exfoliants or very low-concentration AHAs.
- **Frequency:** Every 10 days or as tolerated.
- **Tips:** Look for soothing ingredients like oatmeal or chamomile.

DIY Exfoliating Recipes for Winter

1. **Honey and Sugar Scrub**
   - **Ingredients:** 1 tbsp honey, 1 tsp finely ground sugar.
   - **How to Use:** Gently massage onto damp skin for 1-2 minutes, then rinse with lukewarm water.
2. **Yogurt and Oatmeal Mask**
   - **Ingredients:** 2 tbsp plain yogurt, 1 tbsp ground oats.
   - **How to Use:** Apply as a mask for 10 minutes before massaging and rinsing.
3. **Papaya Enzyme Peel**
   - **Ingredients:** 1 tbsp mashed papaya.

- o **How to Use:** Spread on clean skin, leave for 5-10 minutes, then rinse off.

Common Mistakes to Avoid

1. **Over-Exfoliating**
   - o Can lead to redness, irritation, and a weakened skin barrier.
   - o **Tip:** Always listen to your skin; less is more.
2. **Skipping Sunscreen**
   - o Freshly exfoliated skin is more sensitive to UV damage. Use a broad-spectrum SPF daily.
3. **Using Harsh Products**
   - o Products with high alcohol content or rough scrubbing particles can do more harm than good.
4. **Ignoring Hydration**
   - o Exfoliation can dehydrate the skin if not followed by adequate moisturization.

Signs of Effective Exfoliation

- **Smoother Texture:** No more rough patches or flakes.
- **Enhanced Glow:** Skin appears brighter and more even-toned.
- **Improved Absorption:** Skincare products work more effectively.

- **Comfort:** No tightness, stinging, or irritation post-exfoliation.

The Balance Between Exfoliation and Rest

Remember, exfoliation is not a daily task. Your skin needs time to recover and build resilience between sessions. Pairing exfoliation with nourishing and hydrating routines ensures your winter skincare journey remains balanced and effective.

Conclusion

Day 4 of your 7-day winter skincare challenge has focused on exfoliating gently and effectively, helping your skin glow without compromising its health. The right techniques and products will remove dullness while keeping your skin barrier intact.

Tomorrow, in Chapter 9, we'll explore Day 5—targeting specific skin concerns with treatments and masks tailored to your needs.

***

Day 5 - Targeted Treatments for Winter Skin Concerns

Winter skin issues can vary widely, from redness and irritation to acne and hyperpigmentation. On Day 5 of your winter-proof skincare journey, we focus on addressing specific skin concerns with targeted treatments and masks. By tailoring your skincare routine to your unique needs, you can tackle problem areas effectively while maintaining overall skin health.

Identifying Common Winter Skin Concerns

1. **Dryness and Flakiness**
   - **Cause:** Reduced humidity and exposure to harsh weather.
   - **Solution:** Deeply hydrating treatments with humectants and emollients.
2. **Redness and Sensitivity**
   - **Cause:** A compromised skin barrier and extreme temperature changes.
   - **Solution:** Soothing masks and treatments with anti-inflammatory ingredients.
3. **Breakouts and Congestion**
   - **Cause:** Heavy moisturizers, sweat from layering clothing, and stress.
   - **Solution:** Lightweight treatments with salicylic acid or niacinamide.
4. **Hyperpigmentation and Dullness**

- o **Cause:** Post-inflammatory marks, reduced cell turnover, and UV exposure.
- o **Solution:** Brightening treatments with Vitamin C, AHAs, or retinoids.

Targeted Treatments for Each Concern

Dryness and Flakiness

- **Key Ingredients:** Hyaluronic acid, glycerin, squalane, shea butter.
- **Recommended Products:** Hydrating serums, sheet masks, or sleeping packs.
- **DIY Solution:**
  - o Mix 1 tsp aloe vera gel with 2 drops of squalane oil. Apply as an overnight treatment.

Redness and Sensitivity

- **Key Ingredients:** Centella asiatica, chamomile, calendula, panthenol.
- **Recommended Products:** Barrier-repair creams, calming face masks, or ampoules.
- **DIY Solution:**
  - o Brew chamomile tea and cool it. Soak a cotton pad in the tea and apply it as a compress for 10 minutes.

Breakouts and Congestion

- **Key Ingredients:** Salicylic acid, tea tree oil, niacinamide, bentonite clay.
- **Recommended Products:** Spot treatments, pore-clearing masks, or mattifying moisturizers.
- **DIY Solution:**
  - Create a mask with 1 tbsp bentonite clay and 2 tsp apple cider vinegar. Apply for 10 minutes and rinse.

Hyperpigmentation and Dullness

- **Key Ingredients:** Vitamin C, kojic acid, licorice extract, glycolic acid.
- **Recommended Products:** Brightening serums, peel pads, or overnight exfoliating masks.
- **DIY Solution:**
  - Blend 1 tbsp mashed papaya with 1 tsp lemon juice. Apply as a mask for 5-10 minutes.

How to Incorporate Treatments into Your Routine

1. **Morning Routine**
   - **Focus:** Protect and brighten.
   - Use Vitamin C serums to reduce pigmentation and boost radiance.

- o Apply a lightweight moisturizer followed by SPF to protect against UV rays.

2. **Evening Routine**
   - o **Focus:** Repair and regenerate.
   - o Apply targeted serums after cleansing and toning, followed by a nourishing night cream.

3. **Weekly Additions**
   - o Use masks or intensive treatments 1-2 times a week, depending on your skin's needs.

Winter-Proof Mask Ideas

1. **Hydrating Avocado Mask**
   - o **Ingredients:** 2 tbsp mashed avocado, 1 tsp honey, 1 tsp olive oil.
   - o **How to Use:** Apply for 15 minutes and rinse.

2. **Brightening Yogurt Mask**
   - o **Ingredients:** 2 tbsp plain yogurt, 1 tsp turmeric, 1 tsp lemon juice.
   - o **How to Use:** Leave on for 10 minutes before rinsing.

3. **Soothing Oat Mask**
   - o **Ingredients:** 2 tbsp ground oats, 1 tbsp honey, 1 tbsp rose water.
   - o **How to Use:** Apply for 15 minutes to calm redness and irritation.

4. **Clay Detox Mask**

- o **Ingredients:** 1 tbsp kaolin clay, 1 tsp aloe vera gel, 2 drops tea tree oil.
- o **How to Use:** Leave on for 10 minutes and rinse.

Lifestyle Tips for Addressing Skin Concerns

1. **Hydrate Inside and Out**
   - o Drink plenty of water and consume hydrating foods like cucumbers and oranges.
2. **Manage Stress**
   - o Practice mindfulness, yoga, or meditation to prevent stress-induced breakouts.
3. **Protect Against Environmental Damage**
   - o Wear scarves and gloves to shield your skin from harsh winds and freezing temperatures.
4. **Adjust Your Diet**
   - o Include skin-loving nutrients like omega-3 fatty acids, Vitamin E, and antioxidants.

Tracking Progress and Adjusting Treatments

It's essential to monitor how your skin responds to targeted treatments. Look out for signs of improvement:

1. **Dryness:** Reduced flakiness and tightness.
2. **Redness:** Calmer, more even-toned complexion.
3. **Breakouts:** Fewer pimples or clogged pores.
4. **Pigmentation:** Lightening of dark spots and a brighter overall tone.

If no improvement is seen after 2-3 weeks, consider consulting a dermatologist or switching to different active ingredients.

Conclusion

Day 5 is about addressing your unique skin concerns and personalizing your routine to achieve the best results. Whether you're battling dryness, redness, or pigmentation, the right combination of treatments and masks can help you regain control over your skin's health.

Next, in Chapter 10, we'll focus on Day 6— creating a protective barrier against winter aggressors to lock in all the hard work you've done so far.

***

Day 6 - Creating a Protective Barrier for Winter Skin

Winter weather can be unforgiving, stripping your skin of its natural defenses and leaving it vulnerable to dryness, irritation, and damage. On Day 6 of your 7-day skincare transformation, the focus is on fortifying your skin with a protective barrier. This step ensures that the hydration, nourishment, and treatments you've applied stay locked in, while external aggressors like wind, cold air, and pollution are kept out.

The Importance of a Skin Barrier

The skin barrier, also known as the stratum corneum, is the outermost layer of your skin. It consists of skin cells held together by lipids, much like bricks and mortar. This barrier is essential for:

1. **Retaining Moisture:** Preventing water loss and dehydration.
2. **Blocking Irritants:** Keeping pollutants and allergens at bay.
3. **Maintaining Balance:** Ensuring skin stays smooth and resilient.

A compromised barrier during winter results in dryness, irritation, and an increased risk of sensitivity. Strengthening this barrier is the key to winter-proof skin.

Key Ingredients for Barrier Repair and Protection

1. **Ceramides**
   - Reinforce the skin's lipid layer to lock in moisture.
   - **Found In:** Barrier creams and moisturizers.
2. **Hyaluronic Acid**
   - Draws water into the skin, keeping it plump and hydrated.
   - **Found In:** Hydrating serums and creams.
3. **Squalane**
   - Mimics the skin's natural oils, sealing in hydration without clogging pores.
   - **Found In:** Lightweight oils and moisturizers.
4. **Petrolatum and Shea Butter**
   - Form an occlusive layer to protect against harsh weather.
   - **Found In:** Heavy-duty creams and balms.
5. **Niacinamide**
   - Repairs the skin barrier and reduces redness.
   - **Found In:** Serums and daily moisturizers.

Building Your Winter Skin Shield Routine

Morning Routine

1. **Cleanser:**
   - Use a gentle, non-stripping cleanser to avoid removing essential oils.
2. **Hydrating Serum:**
   - Apply a serum with hyaluronic acid or glycerin to keep skin hydrated.
3. **Moisturizer with Ceramides:**
   - Layer a ceramide-rich cream to strengthen the skin barrier.
4. **Sunscreen:**
   - Don't skip SPF, even in winter! UV rays can still damage your skin.
5. **Optional Step:**
   - Use a facial oil on top of your moisturizer for extra protection against windburn.

Evening Routine

1. **Double Cleansing:**
   - Start with an oil-based cleanser if you wear makeup, followed by a gentle foam or cream cleanser.
2. **Barrier Repair Serum:**
   - Incorporate a serum with niacinamide or peptides for overnight skin restoration.
3. **Thick Night Cream or Balm:**

- o Lock in moisture with a rich cream containing occlusive agents like shea butter or petrolatum.

4. **Optional Step:**
   - o Use a humidifier overnight to keep your skin hydrated while you sleep.

Protective DIY Recipes

1. **Barrier-Boosting Balm**
   - o **Ingredients:** 2 tbsp shea butter, 1 tbsp coconut oil, 1 tsp beeswax.
   - o **How to Use:** Melt ingredients, mix well, and store in a small jar. Apply as needed.
2. **Hydrating Facial Mist**
   - o **Ingredients:** ½ cup rose water, 1 tsp glycerin, 2 drops lavender essential oil.
   - o **How to Use:** Spray on the skin throughout the day for extra hydration.
3. **Overnight Repair Mask**
   - o **Ingredients:** 2 tbsp aloe vera gel, 1 tsp squalane oil, 1 tsp honey.
   - o **How to Use:** Apply a thin layer before bed and rinse off in the morning.

Lifestyle Adjustments for Barrier Protection

1. **Avoid Long, Hot Showers**
   - While tempting in winter, hot water can strip your skin of natural oils. Use lukewarm water instead.
2. **Wear Protective Clothing**
   - Use scarves, gloves, and hats to shield your skin from the elements.
3. **Increase Indoor Humidity**
   - Run a humidifier to counteract the drying effects of indoor heating.
4. **Stay Hydrated**
   - Drink plenty of water and herbal teas to maintain hydration from within.
5. **Choose Fabrics Wisely**
   - Opt for soft, breathable materials like cotton to prevent friction and irritation.

Signs of a Healthy Skin Barrier

1. **Smooth, Plump Texture:** Skin feels soft and supple.
2. **Reduced Sensitivity:** Less redness and irritation.
3. **Improved Hydration Levels:** No tightness or flakiness.
4. **Balanced Oil Production:** Neither overly dry nor excessively oily.

When to Seek Professional Help

If your skin barrier remains compromised despite following a protective routine, consider consulting a dermatologist. Persistent issues like eczema, severe dryness, or unhealed irritation may require prescription treatments such as ceramide-infused ointments or corticosteroids.

Conclusion

Day 6 emphasizes the importance of building a protective shield to ensure your skin thrives despite winter's challenges. By combining barrier-strengthening ingredients, effective skincare practices, and lifestyle adjustments, you can preserve your skin's health and radiance.

In the final chapter, Day 7, we'll bring all the elements together, focusing on maintaining your glow and creating a sustainable skincare routine.

***

Day 7 - Sustaining Your Winter Glow

Congratulations! You've reached Day 7 of your winter skincare journey. By now, your skin should feel more hydrated, smoother, and healthier, even in the harshest weather conditions. The final step focuses on maintaining your winter glow long-term by adopting sustainable habits and creating a balanced skincare routine tailored to your needs.

Reflecting on the Journey

Throughout the past week, you've learned to:

1. **Understand Your Skin's Needs:** Recognize how winter affects your skin and adapt accordingly.
2. **Layer Skincare Products Effectively:** Build routines that prioritize hydration, protection, and repair.
3. **Target Specific Concerns:** Use treatments for dryness, redness, breakouts, and dullness.
4. **Protect Your Skin Barrier:** Strengthen your skin's natural defenses with nourishing ingredients.

These lessons form the foundation for maintaining a radiant complexion year-round.

Creating a Sustainable Winter Skincare Routine

A consistent routine is key to long-term results. Here's how to structure it:

Morning Routine

1. **Cleanse:**
   - Use a gentle cleanser to remove overnight impurities without stripping moisture.
2. **Hydrate:**
   - Apply a hydrating serum with hyaluronic acid or glycerin.
3. **Protect:**
   - Use a ceramide-rich moisturizer and follow with broad-spectrum sunscreen (SPF 30 or higher).
4. **Optional:**
   - Apply a facial oil for added protection if you're spending time outdoors.

Evening Routine

1. **Double Cleanse:**
   - Start with an oil-based cleanser to remove makeup or sunscreen, followed by a mild foaming or cream cleanser.
2. **Treat:**
   - Use serums or creams with active ingredients like niacinamide, peptides, or retinoids to target specific concerns.

3. **Nourish:**
   - Apply a thick moisturizer or sleeping mask to lock in hydration.

Weekly Treatments

1. **Exfoliation:**
   - Use a gentle chemical exfoliant (AHA or BHA) once or twice a week to boost cell turnover.
2. **Hydrating Masks:**
   - Apply a sheet mask or DIY hydrating mask weekly to maintain moisture levels.
3. **Deep Treatments:**
   - Incorporate specialized masks or serums for breakouts, redness, or pigmentation.

Lifestyle Habits for Radiant Skin

1. **Stay Hydrated:**
   - Drink at least 8 glasses of water daily and eat water-rich fruits like oranges and cucumbers.
2. **Prioritize Sleep:**
   - Aim for 7-9 hours of quality sleep each night to allow your skin to repair.
3. **Protect from the Elements:**

- o Wear scarves, hats, and gloves to shield your skin from wind and cold.
4. **Eat Skin-Healthy Foods:**
   - o Include omega-3 fatty acids, antioxidants, and Vitamin E in your diet.
5. **Manage Stress:**
   - o Practice mindfulness, yoga, or meditation to minimize stress-induced skin issues.

Tips for Adapting to Changing Needs

Your skin's requirements may evolve throughout the season. Pay attention to:

1. **Weather Fluctuations:**
   - o Adjust your routine during particularly cold or dry spells by adding richer products.
2. **Skin Responses:**
   - o Reduce active ingredients like retinoids if you notice sensitivity or irritation.
3. **Activity Levels:**
   - o Use lightweight, non-comedogenic products if you're engaging in physical activities.

Emergency Winter Skin Fixes

1. **For Windburn:**
   - Apply aloe vera gel or a barrier repair cream immediately.
2. **For Cracked Lips:**
   - Use a thick, occlusive lip balm with petrolatum or lanolin.
3. **For Flaky Patches:**
   - Gently exfoliate with a lactic acid serum and follow with a rich moisturizer.
4. **For Redness:**
   - Apply a calming mask with ingredients like chamomile or calendula.

Celebrating Progress

Take a moment to appreciate the progress you've made:

- **Improved Texture:** Your skin feels smoother and softer.
- **Hydrated Glow:** A dewy, radiant complexion despite the cold.
- **Reduced Concerns:** Less redness, fewer breakouts, or diminished flakiness.

Maintaining these results requires consistency and mindful adjustments to your routine.

Looking Beyond Winter

As seasons change, so should your skincare routine. Transitioning from winter to spring involves:

1. **Lightening Textures:**
   - Replace heavy creams with lightweight gels or lotions.
2. **Increasing Exfoliation:**
   - Gradually reintroduce stronger exfoliants as your skin tolerates.
3. **Refreshing Your SPF:**
   - Opt for a lightweight sunscreen to accommodate warmer weather.

Conclusion

Winter may pose challenges, but with the right approach, you've proven that healthy, glowing skin is achievable in just seven days. By continuing to prioritize hydration, protection, and care, your skin will remain resilient and radiant no matter the season.

Embrace your winter glow and let it remind you of the power of self-care. Your skin—and your confidence—deserve nothing less.

***

The Role of Nutrition in Skin Health

When it comes to achieving radiant and healthy skin, the phrase "you are what you eat" holds undeniable truth. Nutrition plays a foundational role in maintaining skin health, especially during the winter months when external conditions can strip your skin of its natural vibrancy. This chapter dives into how key nutrients impact skin health and offers practical tips for incorporating them into your diet.

How Nutrition Affects the Skin

The skin is the body's largest organ and a reflection of overall health. Nutrients obtained from food serve as building blocks for skin repair, hydration, and protection against environmental damage. A balanced diet helps to:

1. **Maintain Skin Barrier Integrity:** Essential fatty acids support the lipid layer.
2. **Promote Collagen Production:** Vitamins and proteins aid in skin elasticity and resilience.
3. **Protect Against Oxidative Stress:** Antioxidants neutralize free radicals that cause aging.
4. **Hydrate from Within:** Water-rich foods and electrolytes enhance skin hydration.

Key Nutrients for Skin Health

1. Vitamin A

- **Role:** Promotes cell turnover, reduces dryness, and supports skin repair.
- **Sources:** Sweet potatoes, carrots, spinach, kale, eggs, and liver.

2. Vitamin C

- **Role:** Boosts collagen production, brightens skin, and protects against UV damage.
- **Sources:** Oranges, strawberries, bell peppers, broccoli, and kiwi.

3. Vitamin E

- **Role:** Acts as a potent antioxidant, protecting the skin from oxidative damage.
- **Sources:** Almonds, sunflower seeds, avocados, and olive oil.

4. Zinc

- **Role:** Helps heal skin wounds and reduces inflammation, particularly useful for acne-prone skin.
- **Sources:** Pumpkin seeds, lentils, chickpeas, oysters, and beef.

5. Omega-3 Fatty Acids

- **Role:** Strengthens the skin barrier, reduces inflammation, and combats dryness.

- **Sources:** Salmon, flaxseeds, walnuts, chia seeds, and sardines.

6. Biotin (Vitamin B7)

- **Role:** Supports healthy skin, hair, and nails.
- **Sources:** Eggs, bananas, nuts, and whole grains.

7. Collagen and Protein

- **Role:** Provides structural support to the skin and enhances elasticity.
- **Sources:** Bone broth, chicken, fish, tofu, and legumes.

8. Antioxidants

- **Role:** Neutralize free radicals that accelerate aging and skin damage.
- **Sources:** Blueberries, dark chocolate, green tea, and pomegranates.

9. Water and Electrolytes

- **Role:** Keeps skin hydrated and maintains its plumpness.
- **Sources:** Water, coconut water, cucumbers, and watermelon.

Foods to Avoid for Better Skin

Certain foods can aggravate skin conditions or accelerate aging. Limit the intake of:

1. **Processed Sugars:** Can lead to inflammation and collagen breakdown.
2. **Dairy Products:** May contribute to acne for some individuals.
3. **Fried Foods:** High in unhealthy fats, which can clog pores.
4. **Alcohol:** Dehydrates the skin and disrupts the body's natural detoxification processes.

Sample Meal Plan for Healthy Skin

Breakfast:

- Smoothie with spinach, banana, almond milk, chia seeds, and a handful of berries.
- Whole-grain toast with avocado and a boiled egg.

Lunch:

- Grilled salmon with quinoa and a side of steamed broccoli and carrots.
- A green salad topped with olive oil, sunflower seeds, and roasted sweet potatoes.

Snack:

- Handful of mixed nuts and seeds.
- Green tea and a small piece of dark chocolate.

Dinner:

- Chicken or tofu stir-fry with bell peppers, zucchini, and brown rice.
- Side of kale sautéed in garlic and olive oil.

Dessert:

- Greek yogurt with a drizzle of honey and pomegranate seeds.

Hydration Tips for Winter Skin

1. **Drink Water Consistently:** Aim for at least 8 glasses daily.
2. **Incorporate Herbal Teas:** Chamomile, green tea, or peppermint tea can hydrate and provide antioxidants.
3. **Eat Water-Rich Foods:** Include fruits like oranges, cucumbers, and melons.

The Gut-Skin Connection

A healthy gut contributes to healthy skin. Gut imbalances can manifest as acne, eczema, or rosacea. Support your gut health by:

1. **Including Probiotics:** Found in yogurt, kefir, and fermented foods like kimchi and sauerkraut.

2. **Eating Fiber-Rich Foods:** Promote gut health with fruits, vegetables, and whole grains.
3. **Limiting Processed Foods:** Minimize inflammation by avoiding highly processed items.

Supplements for Skin Health

While a balanced diet should be your primary source of nutrients, supplements can help if deficiencies exist. Consult a healthcare professional before taking:

1. **Fish Oil Capsules:** For omega-3 fatty acids.
2. **Vitamin C or E Tablets:** To boost antioxidant levels.
3. **Collagen Peptides:** To improve skin elasticity and hydration.

Winter Superfoods for Radiant Skin

1. **Sweet Potatoes:** Rich in Vitamin A to promote healthy cell turnover.
2. **Citrus Fruits:** Packed with Vitamin C to brighten skin and fight free radicals.
3. **Avocados:** Full of healthy fats and Vitamin E for moisturized skin.
4. **Nuts and Seeds:** Provide zinc and antioxidants to support barrier repair.

5. **Green Leafy Vegetables:** Loaded with vitamins and minerals for overall skin health.

Conclusion

Nutrition forms the backbone of a successful skincare routine, especially during the winter months. By nourishing your body with skin-loving nutrients and avoiding harmful foods, you can enhance your skin's natural glow from within.

As you move forward in your skincare journey, remember that beauty truly starts on the inside—and your plate is the perfect place to begin.

***

Overcoming Common Winter Skin Issues

Winter can be tough on the skin, often bringing with it a host of problems like dryness, redness, and sensitivity. These issues arise due to cold temperatures, low humidity, and indoor heating, which can strip the skin of moisture and weaken its natural barrier. This chapter delves into the most common winter skin challenges and provides actionable solutions to help you keep your skin healthy and glowing throughout the season.

Common Winter Skin Problems and Their Solutions

1. Dryness and Dehydration

Symptoms:

- Tight, flaky, or rough skin.
- Itchiness and discomfort.

Causes:

- Low humidity in the air.
- Overuse of hot water in showers and cleansing routines.

Solutions:

- **Use a Humidifier:** Add moisture to the air in your home.
- **Switch to a Cream-Based Cleanser:** Avoid foaming cleansers that strip natural oils.
- **Apply a Rich Moisturizer:** Use one containing hyaluronic acid, ceramides, or glycerin.
- **Limit Hot Showers:** Opt for lukewarm water instead.

2. Chapped Lips

Symptoms:

- Cracked, peeling, or sore lips.

Causes:

- Constant exposure to wind and cold.
- Licking lips frequently, which worsens dryness.

Solutions:

- **Apply Lip Balm Regularly:** Look for balms with shea butter, beeswax, or petrolatum.
- **Exfoliate Gently:** Use a soft toothbrush or sugar scrub to remove flakes.
- **Protect Lips Outdoors:** Wear a scarf over your mouth during cold weather.

3. Itchy Skin (Winter Itch)

Symptoms:

- Persistent itchiness, especially on arms, legs, and hands.

Causes:

- Dry air and lack of proper hydration.
- Irritation from woolen clothing.

Solutions:

- **Use Fragrance-Free Products:** Avoid products with harsh chemicals or artificial scents.
- **Apply a Thick Body Lotion:** Use one containing oatmeal or shea butter immediately after bathing.
- **Wear Soft, Breathable Fabrics:** Opt for cotton or moisture-wicking layers under wool.

4. Redness and Sensitivity

Symptoms:

- Red or irritated patches, particularly on cheeks and around the nose.

Causes:

- Cold winds and fluctuating indoor-outdoor temperatures.
- Overuse of exfoliants or active skincare ingredients.

Solutions:

- **Layer a Barrier Cream:** Apply before going outside to shield your skin.
- **Avoid Over-Exfoliation:** Limit exfoliation to once a week.
- **Use Calming Products:** Look for ingredients like chamomile, calendula, or aloe vera.

5. Flaky Scalp and Dandruff

Symptoms:

- White flakes on the scalp and shoulders.
- Itchiness or tightness on the scalp.

Causes:

- Dry indoor air and cold outdoor temperatures.
- Overuse of hot water while washing hair.

Solutions:

- **Use a Moisturizing Shampoo:** Choose one with tea tree oil or zinc pyrithione.
- **Avoid Hot Water:** Wash your hair with lukewarm water.
- **Apply Scalp Treatments:** Use oils like coconut or argan oil for deep hydration.

6. Acne and Breakouts

Symptoms:

- Pimples, blackheads, or whiteheads, often due to heavy skincare products.

Causes:

- Over-moisturizing with rich, comedogenic products.
- Lack of proper cleansing, leading to clogged pores.

Solutions:

- **Use Non-Comedogenic Products:** Opt for lightweight, oil-free moisturizers.
- **Cleanse Thoroughly:** Remove makeup and sunscreen before bed.
- **Spot-Treat Breakouts:** Use salicylic acid or benzoyl peroxide sparingly.

7. Eczema and Psoriasis Flare-Ups

Symptoms:

- Patches of inflamed, itchy, or scaly skin.

Causes:

- Cold weather and dry air exacerbate these chronic conditions.

Solutions:

- **Consult a Dermatologist:** Prescription creams or treatments may be necessary.
- **Use Gentle, Hydrating Products:** Stick to fragrance-free, hypoallergenic options.
- **Moisturize Frequently:** Apply emollients or ointments to affected areas multiple times a day.

Preventive Measures for Winter Skin Care

1. **Hydrate Internally:**
   - Drink plenty of water and consume water-rich fruits and vegetables.
2. **Protect Skin Outdoors:**
   - Use scarves, gloves, and SPF products to shield skin from wind and UV rays.
3. **Use Overnight Masks:**
   - Apply hydrating or barrier-repair masks at night for intensive care.
4. **Follow a Consistent Routine:**
   - Stick to a simple routine with moisturizing and protective products.
5. **Monitor Skin's Needs:**
   - Adjust your skincare routine as your skin's condition changes with the weather.

DIY Remedies for Common Winter Issues

1. **Soothing Oatmeal Bath:**
   - **Ingredients:** 1 cup of colloidal oatmeal.
   - **How to Use:** Add to a warm bath and soak for 15-20 minutes to relieve itchiness.
2. **Lip Scrub:**
   - **Ingredients:** 1 tsp sugar, ½ tsp honey, ½ tsp coconut oil.
   - **How to Use:** Gently massage onto lips, then rinse and apply lip balm.
3. **Scalp Mask:**
   - **Ingredients:** 2 tbsp aloe vera gel, 1 tbsp coconut oil, a few drops of tea tree oil.
   - **How to Use:** Apply to the scalp, leave for 30 minutes, and rinse with a gentle shampoo.

When to Seek Professional Help

If any of these skin issues persist or worsen despite consistent care, it may be time to consult a dermatologist. Conditions like eczema, psoriasis, or severe acne may require prescription treatments or specialized therapies.

Conclusion

Winter skin challenges are common, but with the right knowledge and a proactive approach, you can overcome them effectively. By tailoring your skincare routine and making small lifestyle adjustments, you'll be well-equipped to maintain healthy, comfortable skin throughout the colder months.

In the final chapter, we'll discuss how to integrate all the elements of this book into a cohesive and sustainable skincare routine for the long term.

***

DIY Skincare – Affordable Remedies for Winter

Winter skincare doesn't have to break the bank. With a few simple, natural ingredients, you can create effective remedies to tackle common winter skin issues. This chapter explores a variety of DIY skincare treatments for hydration, exfoliation, and protection, using items readily available in your kitchen or local store. These remedies are not only cost-effective but also free from harsh chemicals, making them suitable for most skin types.

Benefits of DIY Skincare

1. **Cost-Effective:** Uses inexpensive, everyday ingredients.
2. **Customizable:** Tailored to your specific skin needs and preferences.
3. **Natural Ingredients:** Reduces exposure to synthetic additives and irritants.
4. **Eco-Friendly:** Minimal packaging waste and sustainable ingredients.

DIY Remedies for Winter Skincare

1. Moisturizing Face Mask

Purpose: Deeply hydrates and soothes dry, flaky skin.

Ingredients:

- 2 tbsp avocado (mashed)
- 1 tbsp honey
- 1 tsp olive oil

How to Use:

1. Mix the ingredients into a smooth paste.
2. Apply evenly to clean skin.
3. Leave on for 15–20 minutes, then rinse with lukewarm water.

2. Exfoliating Sugar Scrub

Purpose: Removes dead skin cells and enhances skin texture.

Ingredients:

- 2 tbsp brown sugar
- 1 tbsp coconut oil
- ½ tsp vanilla extract (optional for scent)

How to Use:

1. Combine the ingredients in a small bowl.
2. Gently massage onto damp skin in circular motions.
3. Rinse with warm water and pat dry.

3. Lip Balm

Purpose: Heals and protects chapped lips.

Ingredients:

- 1 tbsp beeswax pellets
- 1 tbsp coconut oil
- 1 tbsp shea butter

How to Use:

1. Melt the ingredients together in a double boiler.
2. Pour into a small container and allow to cool.
3. Apply as needed to keep lips soft and moisturized.

4. Oatmeal Bath Soak

Purpose: Relieves itchy, irritated skin and locks in moisture.

Ingredients:

- 1 cup colloidal oatmeal
- ½ cup baking soda
- 10 drops lavender essential oil (optional)

How to Use:

1. Add the mixture to warm bathwater.
2. Soak for 20 minutes, then pat skin dry.

5. Hand and Foot Cream

Purpose: Repairs cracked, rough skin on hands and feet.

Ingredients:

- 2 tbsp shea butter
- 1 tbsp coconut oil
- 1 tsp aloe vera gel

How to Use:

1. Melt the shea butter and coconut oil.
2. Mix in aloe vera gel once cooled.
3. Massage into hands and feet before bed and wear socks overnight.

6. Hydrating Toner

Purpose: Refreshes and hydrates the skin after cleansing.

Ingredients:

- ½ cup rose water
- 1 tsp glycerin
- 2 drops of chamomile essential oil

How to Use:

1. Mix all ingredients in a spray bottle.

2. Mist onto clean skin or apply with a cotton pad.

7. Soothing Eye Mask

Purpose: Reduces puffiness and hydrates the delicate eye area.

Ingredients:

- 2 slices of cucumber
- 1 tbsp aloe vera gel

How to Use:

1. Apply aloe vera gel to the under-eye area.
2. Place cucumber slices over closed eyes.
3. Relax for 10–15 minutes, then rinse gently.

8. Hair Mask for a Flaky Scalp

Purpose: Moisturizes the scalp and reduces dandruff.

Ingredients:

- 2 tbsp yogurt
- 1 tbsp honey
- 1 tsp coconut oil

How to Use:

1. Mix the ingredients thoroughly.
2. Massage onto the scalp and hair.
3. Leave for 30 minutes before rinsing with a gentle shampoo.

9. Gentle Makeup Remover

Purpose: Removes makeup while hydrating the skin.

Ingredients:

- 2 tbsp coconut oil
- 1 tbsp rose water

How to Use:

1. Combine the ingredients in a small jar.
2. Apply to a cotton pad and gently remove makeup.

Tips for DIY Skincare Success

1. **Patch Test First:** Test a small area of skin to avoid reactions.
2. **Store Properly:** Keep DIY products in clean, airtight containers.
3. **Use Fresh Ingredients:** Ensure ingredients are fresh for maximum benefits.
4. **Maintain Hygiene:** Wash hands and tools before preparing any products.

5. **Customize Recipes:** Adjust ingredients based on your skin type and needs.

DIY Skincare Safety Notes

- Avoid using lemon or other acidic ingredients on the skin in winter, as they can increase sensitivity.
- Be cautious with essential oils; they should always be diluted with a carrier oil.
- Discard homemade products if they develop an unusual smell, color, or texture.

Conclusion

DIY skincare remedies are an excellent way to care for your skin during winter while saving money and avoiding harsh chemicals. By incorporating these easy-to-make solutions into your routine, you can address dryness, irritation, and other seasonal concerns with ease.

With a little creativity and a few simple ingredients, you can achieve glowing, healthy skin that feels nourished and cared for throughout the cold months.

*****

Maintaining Your Glow Beyond the 7-Day Challenge

The 7-day winter skincare challenge was designed to jumpstart your journey toward healthier, more radiant skin. However, true skin health requires consistent care and thoughtful habits that extend far beyond a single week. This chapter will guide you on how to sustain your winter glow throughout the season—and even year-round—by building a skincare routine, embracing lifestyle changes, and preparing for seasonal transitions.

Creating a Sustainable Skincare Routine

To maintain the results from the 7-day challenge, it's crucial to establish a consistent skincare regimen tailored to your skin type and concerns.

Morning Routine

1. **Cleanse:** Use a gentle, hydrating cleanser to start your day.
2. **Tone:** Apply a hydrating toner to prep your skin.
3. **Moisturize:** Lock in hydration with a lightweight moisturizer.
4. **Sunscreen:** Always use broad-spectrum SPF, even in winter.

Evening Routine

1. **Double Cleanse:** Remove makeup and impurities with an oil-based cleanser, followed by a water-based cleanser.
2. **Exfoliate:** Use a chemical exfoliant 1–2 times a week to maintain smooth skin.
3. **Serum:** Apply a nourishing serum with ingredients like hyaluronic acid or niacinamide.
4. **Night Cream:** Seal in moisture with a richer cream or sleeping mask.

Lifestyle Changes to Support Skin Health

1. **Stay Hydrated:**
   - Drink at least 8 glasses of water daily to maintain skin hydration.
   - Herbal teas and soups are excellent winter-friendly options.
2. **Eat a Balanced Diet:**
   - Focus on foods rich in omega-3 fatty acids, vitamin E, and antioxidants.
   - Include healthy fats like avocados, nuts, and fish in your diet.
3. **Prioritize Sleep:**
   - Aim for 7–9 hours of quality sleep to support skin repair and regeneration.
   - Use a silk or satin pillowcase to reduce friction and prevent irritation.

4. **Manage Stress:**
   o Practice mindfulness, meditation, or yoga to reduce stress-related skin issues.
   o Engage in hobbies or activities that bring you joy.
5. **Stay Active:**
   o Regular exercise improves blood circulation, delivering oxygen and nutrients to the skin.
   o Choose indoor workouts during extreme weather to avoid harsh conditions.

Adjusting for Seasonal Transitions

As the seasons change, so do your skin's needs. Adapting your skincare routine ensures that your skin remains balanced and healthy year-round.

1. **Spring:**
   o Transition to lighter moisturizers as humidity increases.
   o Focus on gentle exfoliation to remove winter buildup.
2. **Summer:**
   o Prioritize sunscreen and oil-free products to combat heat and UV exposure.
   o Hydrating mists can help refresh your skin throughout the day.
3. **Fall:**

- o Start incorporating richer moisturizers and serums to prepare for colder weather.
- o Repair summer damage with antioxidants like vitamin C.

4. **Winter:**
- o Return to the strategies from the 7-day challenge: richer creams, barrier repair, and deep hydration.
- o Avoid harsh cleansers and over-exfoliating to prevent dryness.

Maintaining Consistency and Motivation

1. **Track Your Progress:**
- o Keep a journal or take weekly photos to monitor changes in your skin.
2. **Simplify Your Routine:**
- o Avoid overloading your regimen with too many products. Stick to essentials that work for your skin.
3. **Reward Yourself:**
- o Treat yourself to a professional facial or new skincare product after reaching milestones.
4. **Learn and Adapt:**
- o Stay informed about your skin type and how it reacts to different seasons and products.
- o Be open to tweaking your routine based on your skin's needs.

Holistic Practices for Long-Term Glow

1. **Skincare from Within:**
   - Supplements like fish oil, collagen, and probiotics can complement your routine.
   - Always consult with a healthcare professional before starting supplements.
2. **Detoxify:**
   - Periodically detox your skin with clay masks to remove impurities.
3. **Pamper Your Skin:**
   - Schedule regular at-home spa days to reinforce the benefits of your routine.
4. **Build a Ritual:**
   - Treat your skincare routine as a moment of self-care and relaxation.

Tools to Support Your Glow

1. **Invest in Skincare Tools:**
   - Use tools like facial rollers, gua sha stones, or LED light therapy devices to enhance your routine.
2. **Embrace Technology:**
   - Apps for tracking your skincare routine and reminders can help you stay consistent.
3. **Create a Dedicated Space:**

- o Set up a calming area for your skincare regimen to make it feel luxurious and special.

***

Conclusion

Maintaining your glow beyond the 7-day challenge is about embracing consistent habits, making thoughtful lifestyle choices, and adjusting your routine with the seasons. By integrating these practices into your daily life, you'll not only preserve your winter glow but also cultivate a foundation for long-term skin health.

Remember, skincare is a journey, not a destination. Celebrate the progress you've made and continue nurturing your skin with care and patience. With these strategies, you'll carry your radiant glow through every season and into the future.

***

Your skincare journey doesn't end here. How can we help you, please leave a review?

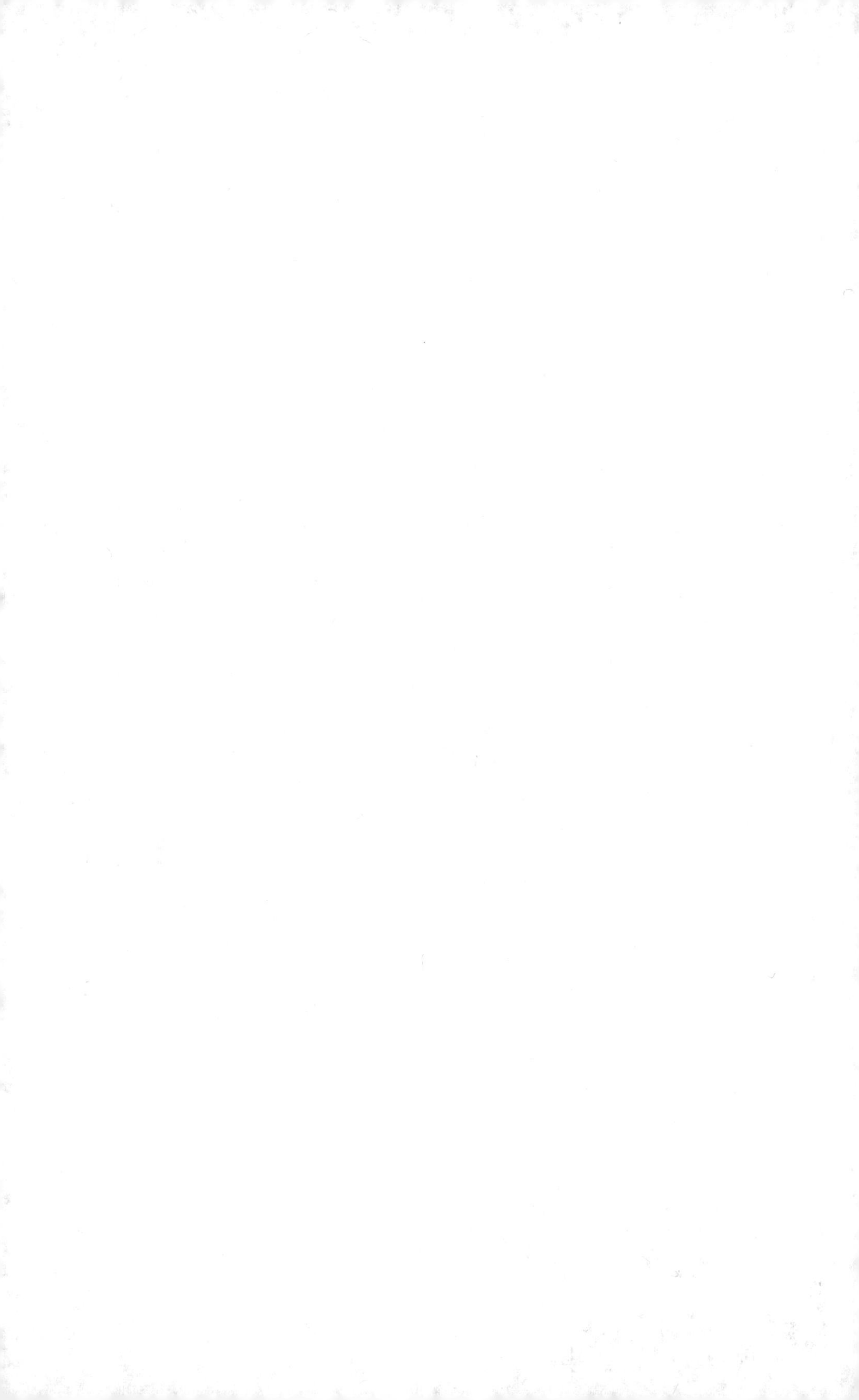